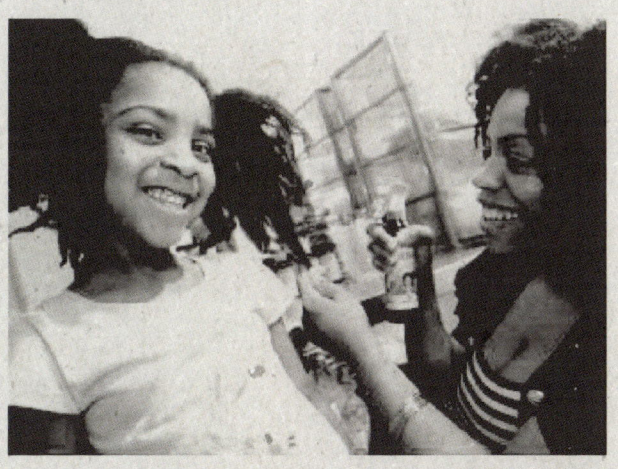

I hope that this book will make many other little girls learn to love their hair just as I helped you to! There is no better gift from a Mother to child, than the gift of loving yourself naturally- and having the confidence to reach for your dreams!

Hair love is priceless.

Hairducation is Power!

Copyright © 2015 by Salem A. Wynter

All rights reserved.

Cover design by A Rhose

Book design by A Rhose

No part of this book may be reproduced in any form or by any electronic or mechanical means including information storage and retrieval systems, without permission in writing from the author. The only exception is by a reviewer, who may quote short excerpts in a review.

This book is a guide based on personal experience and the professional study of haircare.   Disclaimer: Seek professional assistance if deemed necessary.

Visit my website at www.root2tip.com or www.hairducation.org.uk

Printed in EUROPE

First Printing: July 2015

HAIRDUCATION ACADEMY

ISBN-13: 978-1514781814
ISBN-10: 1514781816

CONTENT

1. Introduction
About the writer: My Story!

2. Different Hair Types
Types 3a - 4z: Why it makes life easier if you had an idea of such!

3. Hair Confidence
Why it is so important for your child to love their hair for inner confidence and self esteem.

4. Splish, Splash, Splosh
It's time to wash - Tantrum free hair wash days!

5. Knot on my watch
Detangling 101 - Keep knots and matting away!

6. Frizz Fairy!
How to avoid but also embrace the Frizzy fairy!

7. Sandwich
Say bye to dry hair with our fool-proof 'Sandwich' moisture method!

8. Say no to relaxer!
Why straightening chemicals are bad for curly/Afro kids

9. Conditioners
Truly a curls best friend!

10. Simple Style Guide
Twists / Plaits Instructions

11. Product Guide
Finding the right product range!

12. Invest
Essential Items to invest in for your child's hair

13. FAQ's
FAQ's on everything kiddy hair

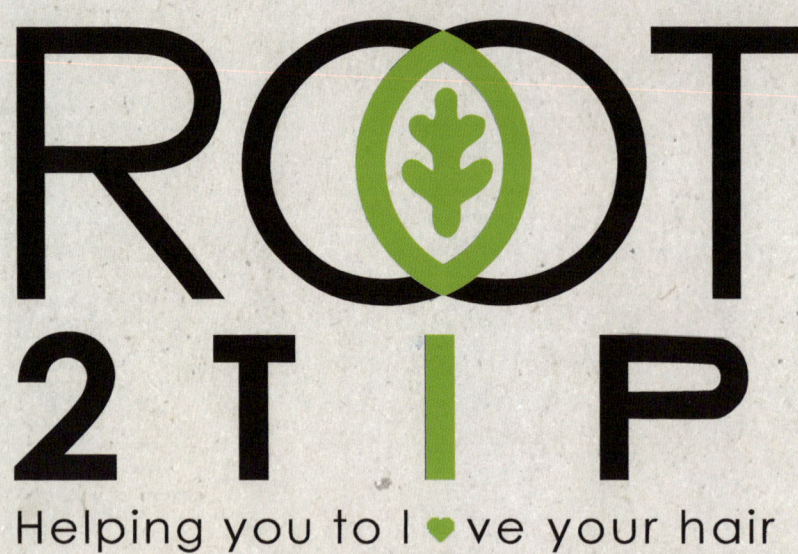

Thank-you for purchasing this book today, you are one-step closer to eliminating stressful hair days with your child at home! Happy hair days are possible with a little hairducation.

This Hair care guide has been lovingly written to give you the basic Hairducation needed to successfully manage your child's unique, beautiful Mixed race or Afro hair texture and everything in between.

If you are a new mom and you have a mixed race child and you are nervous about how to best care for their curls, be confident this guide will gently point you in the right direction!

We will go through How to wash the hair- (with no tears!), dealing with knots, frizz and tangles plus simple styles for those who cannot braid or twist. There is also a FAQ's section of the most common asked questions in relation to kids with kinks and curls!

We also discuss why your child must be taught to have hair confidence especially true for children in care or if they have been newly adopted.

Hair is very powerful so by having the right Hairducation tailored to your child's hair type you will be able to teach your child how to love themselves naturally and pass on great hairducation tools and techniques.

About the writer: My story!

As the founder of the natural hair-are company ROOT2TiP started with a loan of £2000 from the Princes trust and the HAIRDUCATION Academy in London, I have devoted my life to helping people to love and understand their hair through Hairducation. It's more than just hair care to me, it's about life! As an expert in Hairducation I have written multiple articles for high-street magazines such as Pride, Black Beauty & Hair and my brand has been featured in Cosmopolitan magazine. We also conduct Hairducation workshops all over Europe.

Hair Obsession

I became obsessed with mixed race and Afro children's hair when my daughter was little. My first child was born with 6 food allergies and chronic eczema. As a result I immediately knew that whatever I used on her hair, that was very thick and fizzy as a toddler, had to be natural! Having scoured my local hair product retailer for a solution I was dumbfounded to find nothing was suitable, all the products contained harmful chemicals. So I decided to research and teach myself how to make my own natural products in addition how to best care for her hair. 'As her hair flourished under my hair routine other parents would request my help and I often spent hours giving out hair tips for mums in the supermarket, street and school playground! I loved to help.'

Hair Workshops

In 2010 I decided to reach out to foster/Adoption agencies and market my Hairducation services to them as I knew the need for help was a reality. They were so grateful for the help, as one parent quoted "this workshop has been the answer to my prayers!" I have been running workshops for Foster carers, adoptive and biological parents of children ever since, we even did the first ever workshop of its kind in Milan, Italy- that was historical. Mixed race and Afro hair is very unique and if you are a parent whom has never come into contact with this beautiful hair texture the maintenance of it can be very difficult at first, as you will have realised it is not simply wash & go hair!

Passion

Although I have created a range of products that are sold globally and have helped so many parents realise the true beauty of their children's hair- my passion first and foremost will always be Hairducation! You can have the best product in the world but unless you have hairducation you may not know what to do with it!

DIFFERENT HAIR TYPES

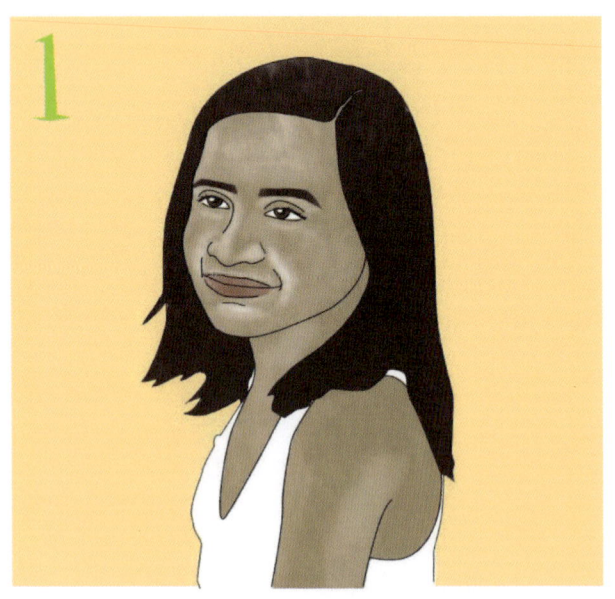
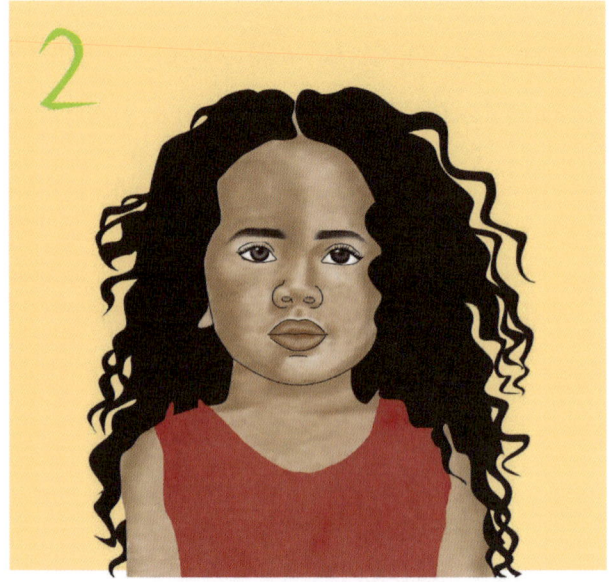
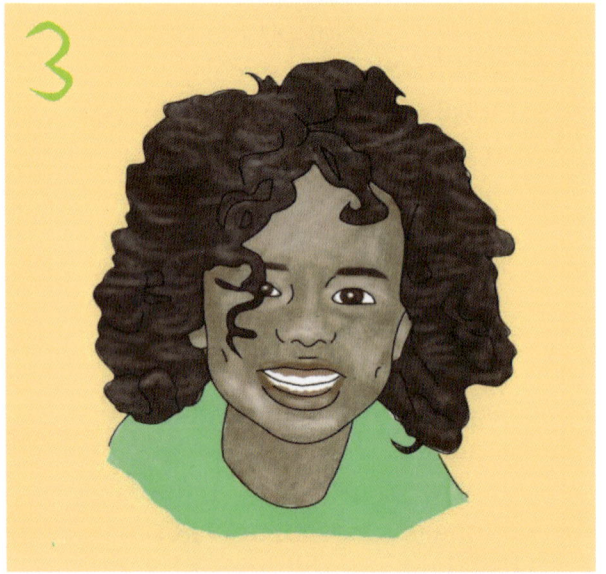
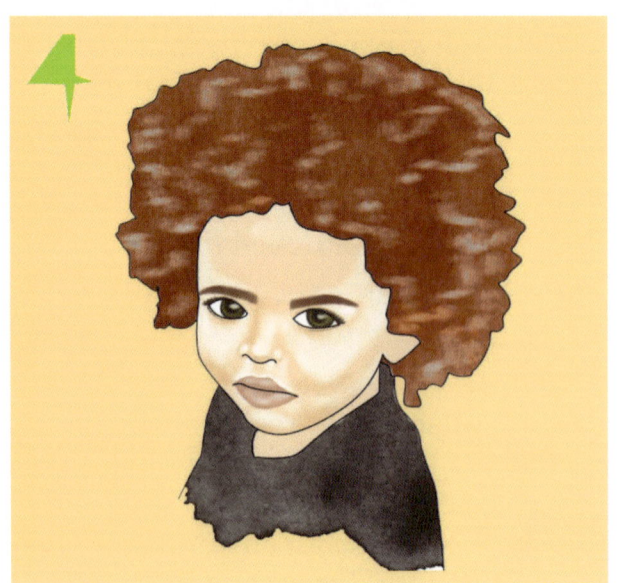

What is your child's hair type?

1 Straight Hair

2 Wavy Hair

3 Curly Hair
3c Type looser curls / 3b tighter spiral curls / 3c kinky/curly

4 Kinky / Afro Hair
4a z-shaped curls, coiled / 4b spiral tight coils, fine, wiry, and densely packed

2 siblings different hair textures!

If you have more than one child you look after you may have noticed that even if they are siblings or from a similar or the same racial background, no two heads of hair are the same! You may have one child with very thick tightly coiled hair strands, which when washed shrinks up to the scalp! And another who may be a sibling with a head full of frizzy but looser s-shaped curls, that when washed hang long and stretched out!

Makes life easy!

This is where knowing your child's hair type comes into play. By understanding and having a vague idea of **your child's hair type you are able to choose products that will maintain the hair more effectively, and also** you will know what works for one type of head may not produce the same results in the second!

Slightly Confused?

If you are now feeling a bit confused- don't worry- its only meant to give you a vague idea of the **difference in hair types, the key thing is choosing products that make life easier for you and the child.**

The nature of: Curly/afro hair makes it very dry, so it needs be moisturised daily, once the correct **moisture level is attained the hair becomes a pleasure to deal with!**

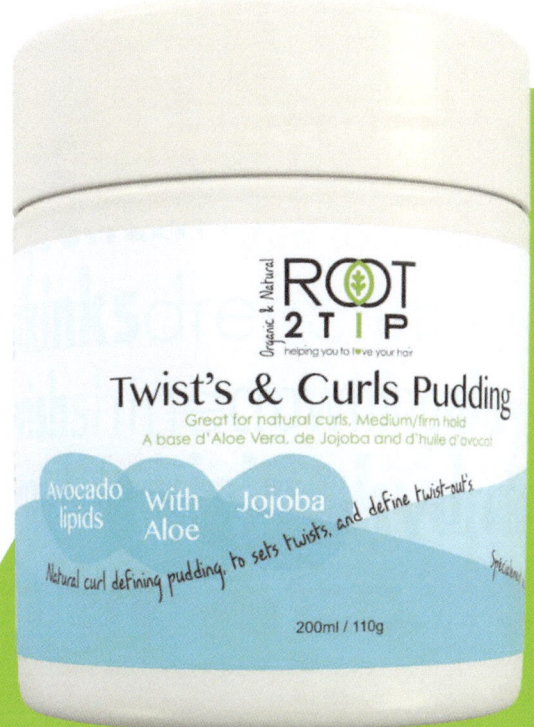

Product choice:

The general rule of thumb is the more curly/kinki the hair the more moisture it will crave.

Type 3 hair (curly) likes to be conditioned regularly and moisturised with products that define the curl and tame the frizz, like moisture rich cream or gel products.

Type 4 hair (Kinki) likes to be Deep conditioned regularly and moisturised with heavier products that eliminate dryness- like hair butters and rich cremes.

HAIR

- Children need to be taught to love themselves especially when placed in foster environments- teaching them about their individuality means giving them an appreciation of their hair and the uniqueness of it.

- If you are a carer who does not share the same racial background of the child you look after- you have to work even harder to understand the uniqueness of your child's hair and skin, this shows the child you have a vested interest in them.

- Children take pride in their appearance from aged 3 upwards, they like to look in the mirror and they like to play with their hair! Once your child's hair is well looked after, the beauty of it will be clear for them to see and over time- learn to love.

- Teaching a child about the uniqueness of their appearance can have a long-lasting positive effect. The child may feel like he/she does not fit in, especially if they are amongst other people who do not resemble them.

- If you are not black / mixed yourself then it is very important to understand that how you address, approach and care for your child/ren's hair, will ultimately have a significant imp at on how your child/ren will perceive themselves, their race, and your view of the racial differences you share.

- It is all too easy to mistakenly cause a child to feel 'inferior' or 'less than' simply because we avoid handling or neglect their hair - which is- in this society, a primary element in defining "beauty."

- Invest the time in learning about your child's uniqueness. Invest the time in finding hair products that compliment and make life easy to maintain their specific texture of hair.

- Hair is meant to be fun, don't make it a chore, make the haircare ritual a bonding time between you.

- Lastly, invest the time in getting your child to love themselves and the hair they are born with, avoiding harsh straightening chemicals no matter the Kink, Coil or Curl.

Why it is so important for your child to love their hair for inner confidence and self esteem?

CONFIDENCE

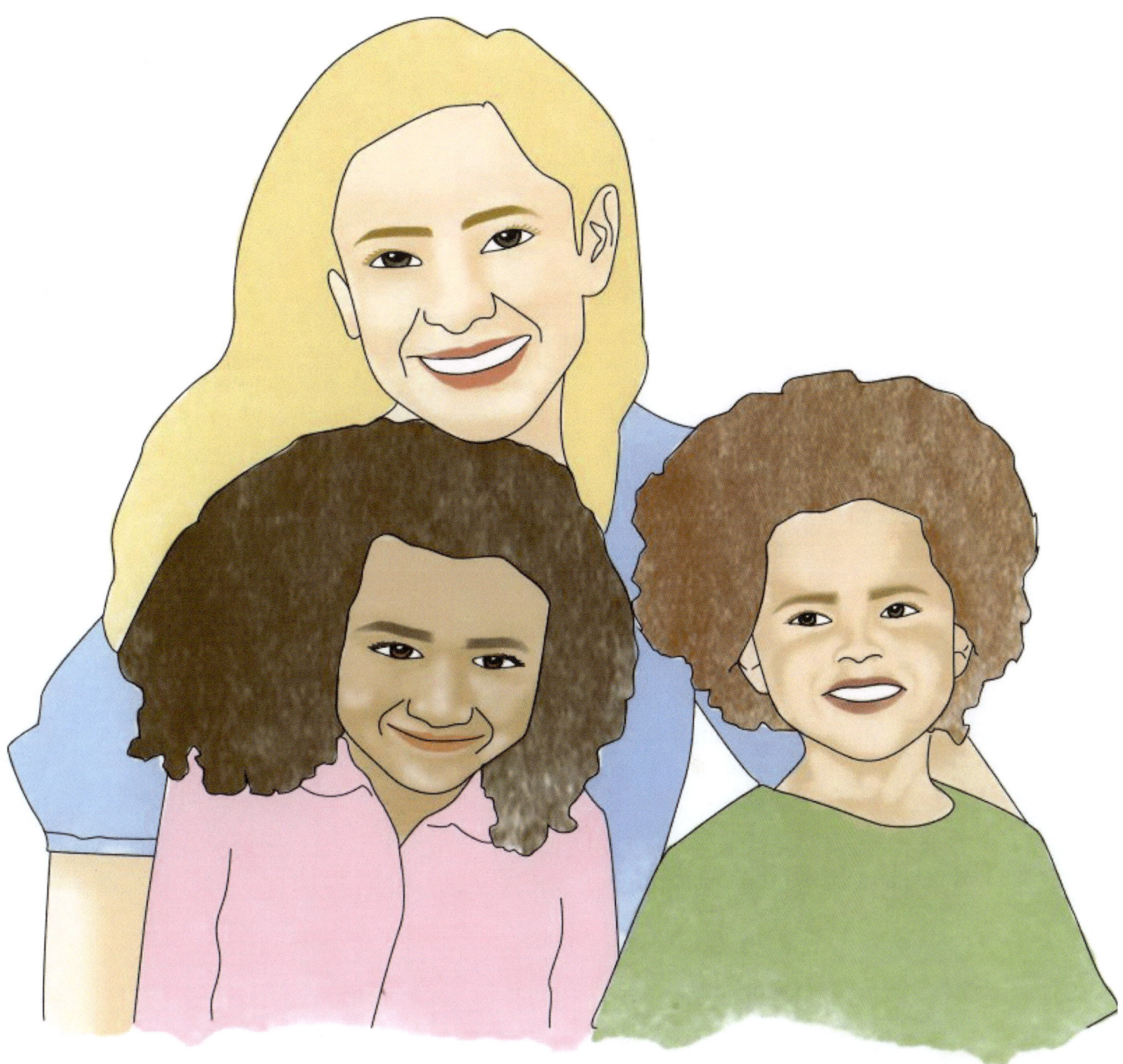

SPLISH, SPLASH SPLOSH!

IT'S WASH TIME!

Hairwash days with Curly and Afro hair!

You may have found already through past experience that washing Curly/Afro hair is a very different experience to washing straight hair!

There is no such thing as a wash & go! By that I mean- it's not a quick experience as the nature of curly/afro hair does not permit this! However there are things you can do to make this experience as trauma free as possible for you and your child.

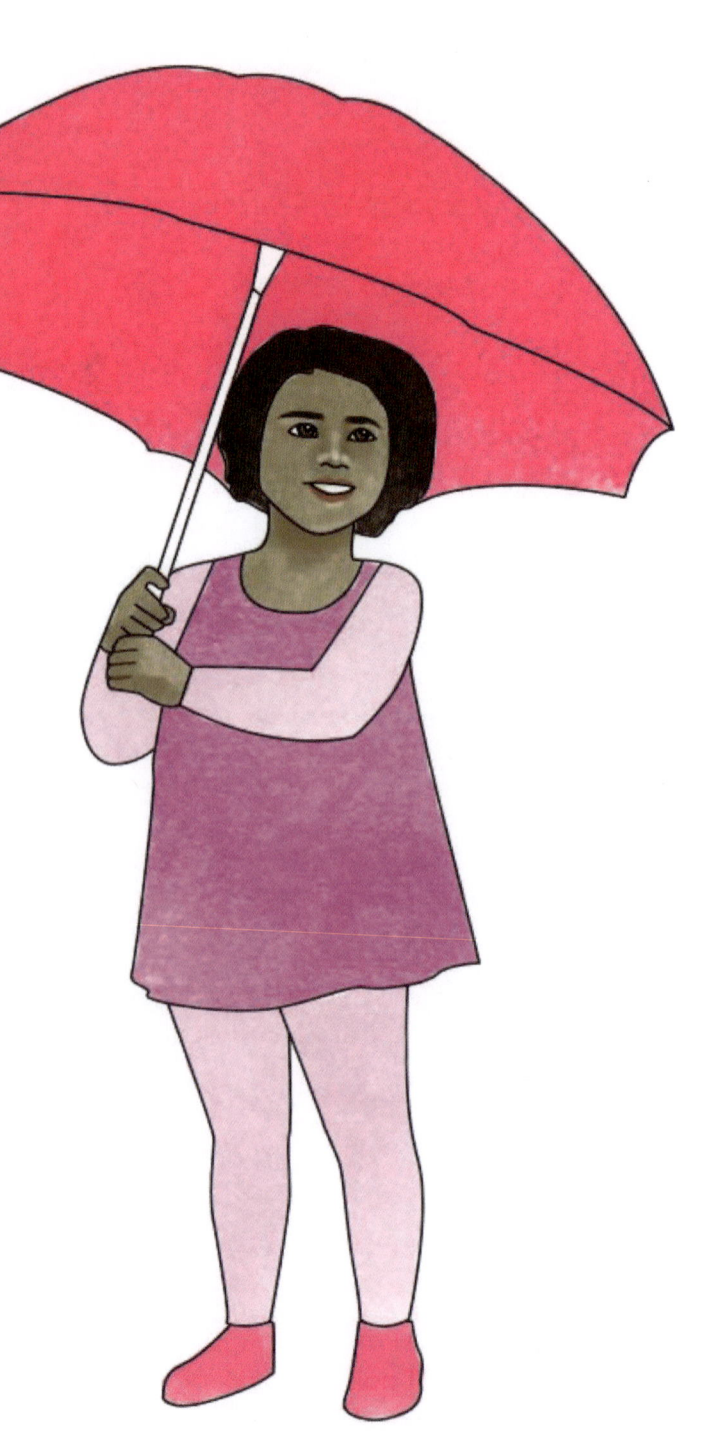

TOP tips for tear free hair washing

1. DETANGLE, DETANGLE, DETANGLE! I say this 3 times because I mean it! Before you add any water or shampoo to the child's hair, spend an hour or so detangling the hair in 4-8 sections from root2tip. (Use the honey rain juice detangler to help you).

2. If you have ever made the error of washing tangled hair- you have my sympathy- water multiplies tangles and knots and that can mean tears, tantrums and time!

3. If the hair is long enough, section the hair into 4, 6 or 8 loose plaits. If you are not good at plaiting, use gentle metal free 'banding' bands to secure the hair in the detangled sections.

4. The hair must stay in these sections as you wash it allowing you to deal with each section at your own pace and avoiding the hair tangling when wet.
Rinse the hair thoroughly with lukewarm water, then apply a small amount of shampoo in the palm of your hands and rub together.

5. Next apply the shampoo to the child's scalp only! Using your fingertips, gently massage it into the scalp. Do not apply it to the length of the hair. Remember curly/afro hair is very dry so it needs to retain as much of its natural oils as possible.

6. As the shampoo is rinsed from the scalp it will gently cleanse the length of the hair, without being too drying.

Sal's tip:

"Try to keep shampoo wash-days to a minimum of once a fortnight. Afro/curly hair must not be stripped of its natural oils as it leads to dry brittle hair that easily breaks and tangles. Conditioner cleanses the hair and scalp just as well as a shampoo- Co-wash more frequently. (See the Conditioner tips)"

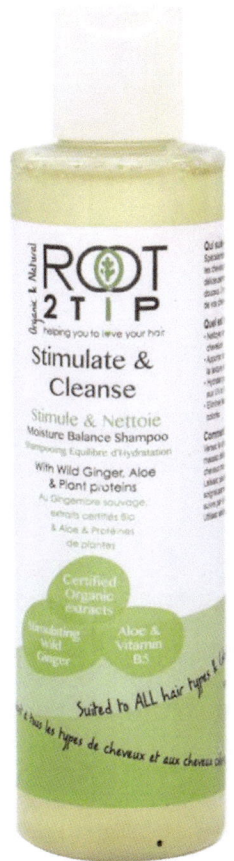

Shampoo Guide:

When it comes to choosing a shampoo for curly/afro hair it should be as mild as possible. Using a regular shampoo designed for straight hair will more than likely leave the hair in a tangled mess

A common cleansing ingredient found in most shampoos is Sodium lauryl/laureth sulphate (SLS), this ingredient when combined with curly/afro hair is like oil and water- they simply do not mix!

Q: So what shampoo is best for curls and afro hair?

You need to use a shampoo that is mild in formulation, look for shampoos that are SLS FREE. SLS means (Sodium lauryl/Laureth sulfate) this ingredient strips the hair dry and it's a cheap cleanser found in most commercial shampoo- (check yours in the bathroom now!)

Instead opt for organic or natural shampoos, milder in formulation they leave hair clean but not stripped dry, which can lead to tangles!

KNOT ON

Firstly, please appreciate that knots and curly/afro hair textures go hand-in-hand like milk and cookies!

HAIR SCIENCE

The unique texture of curly hair lends itself to knotting much more than it does with straight hair. Curls and Kinks that are present in the strands of your childs hair will entwine around each other, which when pulled upon become big knots and single strand knots.

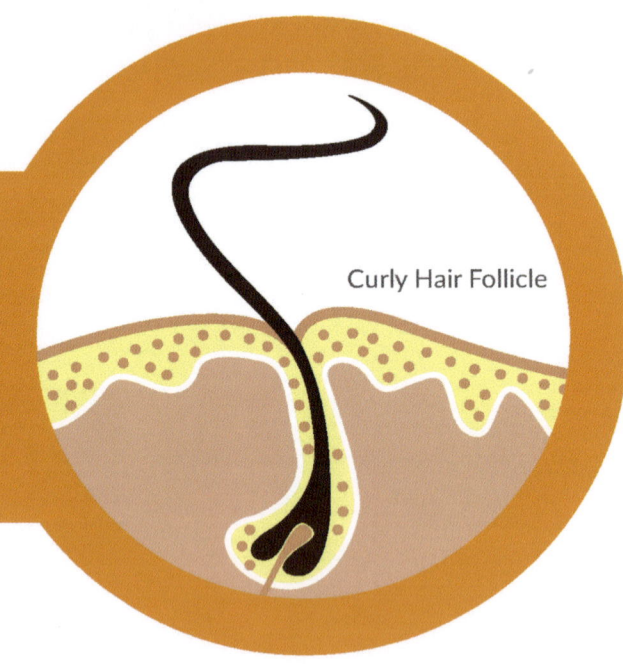
Curly Hair Follicle

Sal's tip:

"The hair needs to be slippery for the knot to loosen without hair damage!"

How to avoid the dreaded hair knots on your watch!

By detangling the hair prior to styling you will lessen the chance of the hair becoming knotted in the first place.

Never sleep with the hair loose if possible. Either braid it into to loose braids or put it into a loose ponytail.

On shorter hair keep the hair in smaller twists that you deal with in sections when taking them down.

MY WATCH

How-to Un-knot your child's hair

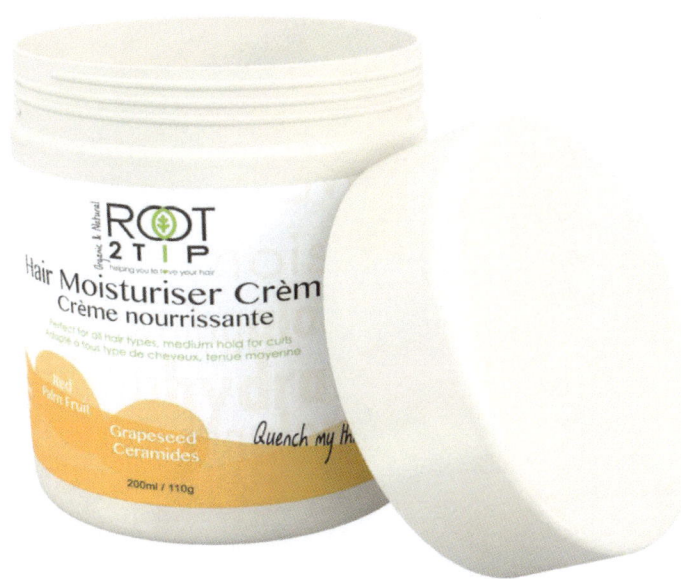

- Apply our curly crème or twurly butter to the ends of hair to prevent knots.

- Never Brush or comb tangled hair- this will increase knots

- Never wash tangled hair- this will multiply knots!

- Keep hair styled in loose twists, banding or single braids to avoid knots.

- If your child has kinky or tight curls the hair will be more prone to knots so if the hair is left out set the hair in a twist out as opposed to a big afro that is likely to tangle and lead to knots. (see styling page)

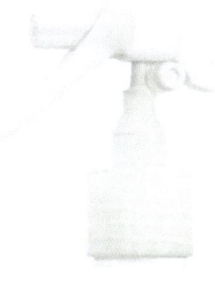

- Spray the hair with our Honey-rain juice detangler- (unrivalled!)

- If you have no products at home, reach for the olive oil in the kitchen, extra virgin is best, saturate knotted hair with it, then wait.

- After a few seconds, hold the knot in between you thumb and midi-finger. With your loose hand gently pull strands out of the knot in an upward action (like pulling straws out of a box.)

- Continue to pull upwards gently strand-by strand. Take your time to avoid breakage.

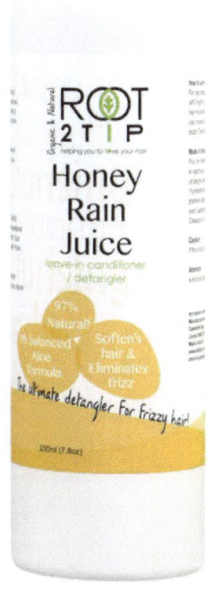

FRIZZ FAIRY

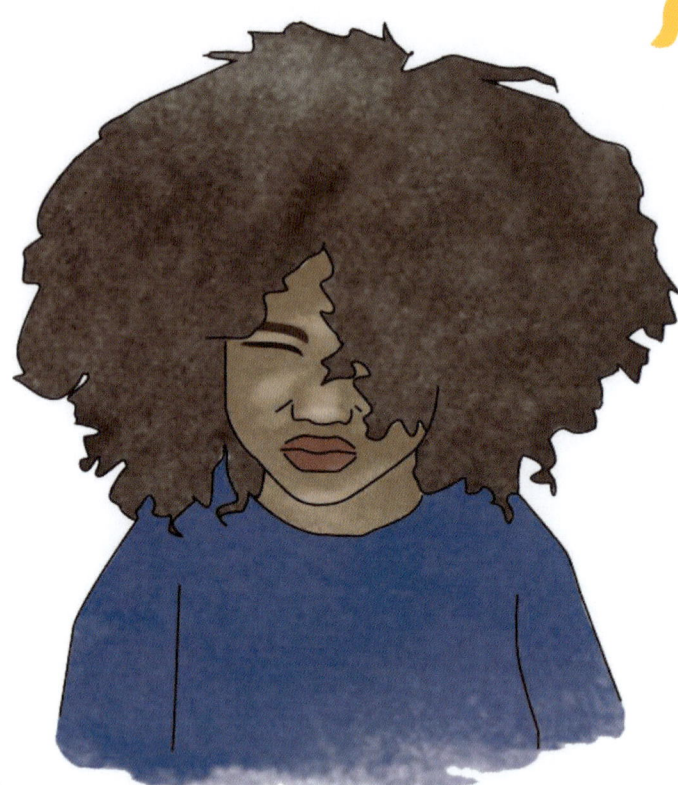

What is Frizzy hair?

Children with naturally curly and Afro hair textures are prone to having frizzy hair due to the unique texture of their hair- from very early on make it a fun thing not a **negative!**

Frizz is generally seen as BAD! In your home make it good as it goes with the territory when you are born with natural curls or afro hair.

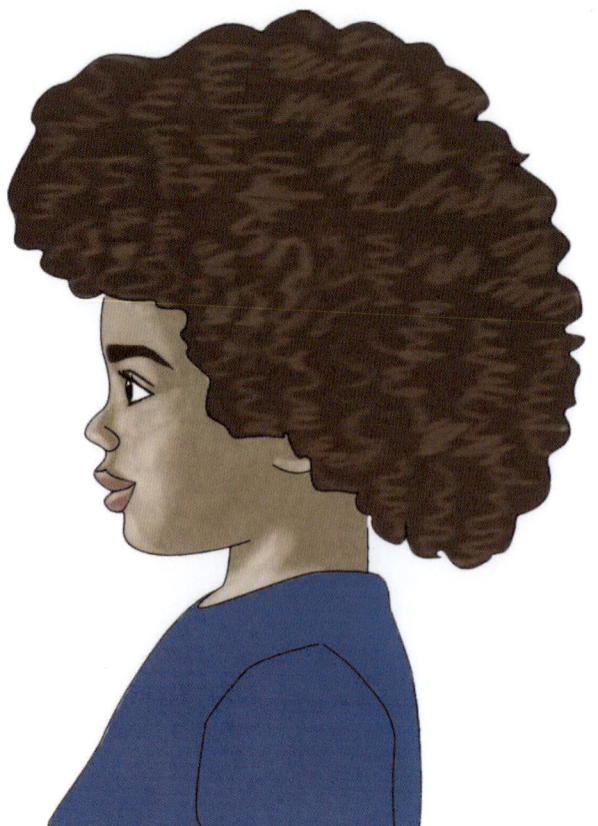

Taming Frizz

The best way to tame frizz is to moisturise your child's hair when it's wet so the **strands and cuticles will lay flat and as the** hair dries it stays that way.

Frizz gets much worse when the hair is lacking in moisture! Or when you go into a humid environment.

How-to moisturise to limit frizz:

1 Co wash your child's hair with our cooler2cowash conditioner, this will smoothe down the strands and leave a film of moisture on the hair even when its rinsed away.

2 In sections spray the Honey rain juice onto damp hair, smooth in the hair from Root to tip.

3 Finally use one of our moisturisers either the Sunlight curl crème or on very thick hair, or the Heavens Hair Milk on fine wavy hair to lock moisture into the hair strands, smoothe, define curls and add lasting hydration.

4 By following this routine you will avoid the frizzy fairy in the morning as the hair is moisturised effectively, the hair will not swell and start to frizz.

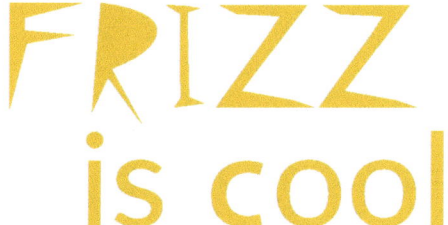

However it's important for your child to embrace every characteristic of their hair very early on for hair confidence- so please teach them how to!

Help your child to love their unique hair by introducing the 'Frizz Fairy'

By making something usually seen as negative into a positive fun experience, your child will be more accepting of it also. It will make hair confidence easier to obtain. The Frizz Fairy is your way of teaching your child about their hair texture and making it FUN!

We want children to say. 'The Frizz fairy always comes out to play with my hair when its dry or not been moisturised yet! By doing so the child is now in control and can then learn how to moisturise their hair properly- Hairducation is Power!

SANDWICH
How to Moisturise kiddy Curls & Afro hair properly!

You may recall me saying earlier that Afro and Mixed curly hair types are almost always dry! But Why?

Without being too scientific- unlike straight hair that uses the natural scalp sebum(oil) to keep the strands hydrated, the curls and kinks in Afro or Curly hair strands mean the sebum cannot hydrate this hair type in the same way! So this means manual moisture is a must!

So How do I moisturise and How often?

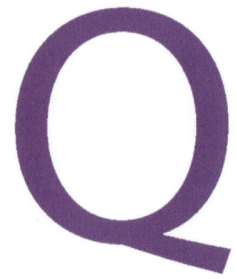

The importance of moisturising:

Moisturising your child's hair should be a daily ritual. (Just like brushing your child's teeth-). Afro/mixed hair types need moisture in order to remain healthy, supple and retain hair growth. (One of the key factors in not seeing hair growth is DRY HAIR)

A sign of healthy moisturised hair is the springiness of it. If you wet your child's hair and then pull a strand of it and it springs back up without breaking, the hair is healthy as it has elasticity. Dry hair breaks at the touch!

*However if your child does not have hair that shrinks up like coils, kinks and some curls, you can tell it's healthy by the smoothness of the waves and feel of it.

The key to effective moisturising is to lock-in the HYDRATION daily!

How and when to moisturise?

The optimum time to moisturise is when your child's hair is damp from washing; if you add your moisturiser on damp hair and in the correct sandwich moisture method (as explained later), the hair will dry naturally and the yummy moisture will be sealed into the strands.

How-often should I moisturise?

Either moisturise your child's hair in the morning before school/nursery or in the evening before bedtime- aim for at least 1 x a day.

If you are moisturising dry hair, or damp hair as explained before this clever 'sandwich layered approach' to moisture as described below will be the answer to your 'dry hair prayers!

> Sal say's:
> **Curls & Afro hair will reflect shine and have great movement irrespective of length if it is well moisturised**

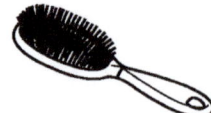

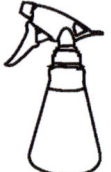

Sal say's:
{Sal say's the correct level of moisture it will enhance the beauty of your child's hair and define curls naturally}

Just to reiterate: Curly, Frizzy and Afro Hair textures tend to be very dry and drink moisture! One moisturiser product alone may not be enough to fully hydrate curly or kinky afro hair- so we have created a sandwich layered way of applying your moisturiser that will give you great results with your child's hair!

The Sandwich Moisture Method

Step 1
Spray Hair with our Honey Rain Juice leave in conditioner- this is a water based product so it makes hair damp and is the first layer in your sandwich.

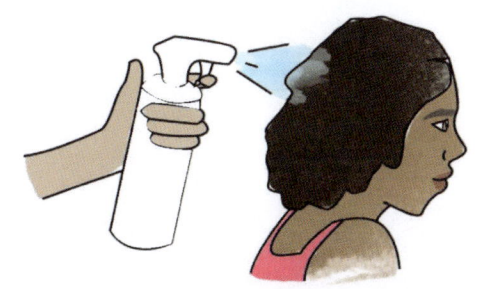

Step 2
Apply a light crème product to seal in more moisture, use our Heaven's hair milk/Sunlight Curl crème and hair is left silky (not greasy) with curls/waves being defined...this is the middle of your sandwich!

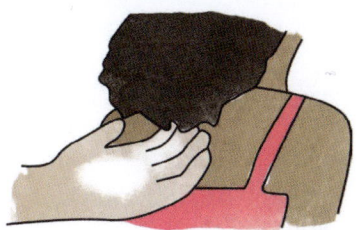

Step 3
To finish off... apply a heavy butter crème like our Vanilla-Sun Twurly butter to seal in all of that yummy natural moisture. This final heavy moisturiser places a shield around the hair that prevents moisture from escaping and defines curls with a lasting shine and hydration.

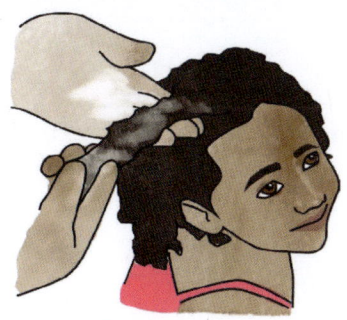

The right hair products and technique changes dry knotty hair into soft bouncy shiny hair in seconds! This is a simple but fool-proof method I have used for years to maintain moisture in my children's hair. The effects will often last for more than 72 hours. It works on every hair texture too- Genius!

Can I use one product only?
Yes you can if the hair is quite fine, or wavy. I would recommend applying your moisturiser of choice on damp hair as described above for best results. Try the Heaven's Hair milk or Twurly butter/ Sunlight Curl Crème as your solo product of choice.

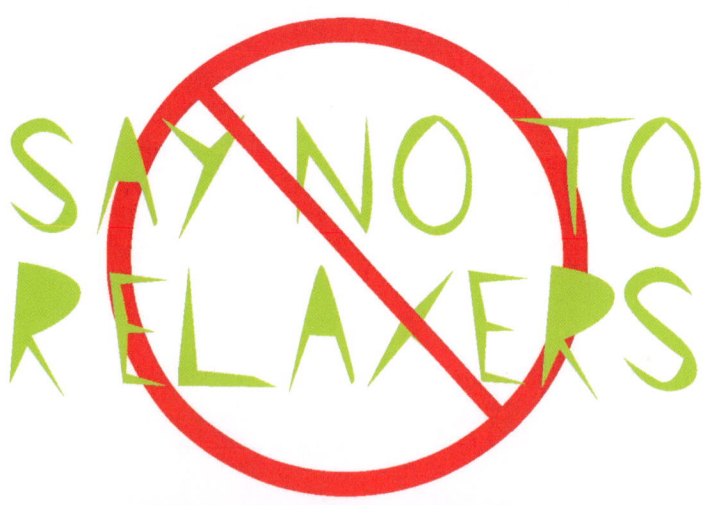

What is a relaxer?

'A relaxer is a chemical cream applied to curly/afro hair to straighten it. The active ingredients in a relaxer are also found in your Drain Cleaner! Yes really!'

If you have a blocked drain you will be relying on the Sodium Hydroxide to clear away the blocked grime. This dangerous chemical is also found in a shop bought relaxers that are applied to children's and teens hair and scalp.

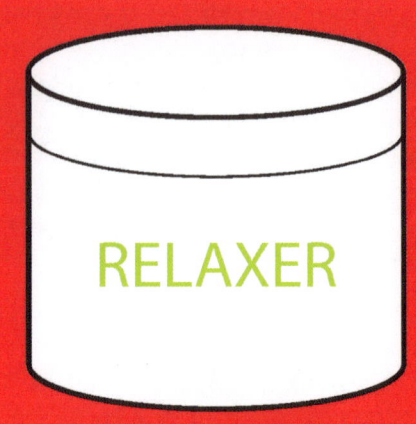

How do relaxers and texturisers work?

Sal says:
"SAY NO TO RELAXER, They are not a *quick fix*"

Relaxers/texturisers work by breaking down protein bonds within the hair strands, the hair is made much weaker due to this. You are then tasked to replace that protein loss and moisture the relaxer has taken away.

Most parents fail to do this effectively- this often results in breakage and dry lifeless hair within 2-3 months of the application.

Relaxers are bad for children's hair for the following reasons:

- Once relaxed hair is weakened by 70%
- Hair will look lifeless, flat and become very dry
- The 'kiddy relaxers' although pictured with a pretty child on the box which is bright and fun - contain the same dangerous chemicals as found in an adult relaxer.
- Relaxer crème can also blindness if it gets into the eyes!
- Once the hair is relaxed it cannot be reversed - removal is via a haircut!
- Relaxing a child's hair can damage their scalps for life as the scalp is young and not yet mature

The hairdresser says
"Relax her hair!"

If you are struggling and you take your child to a hairdresser who advises a relaxer chemical treatment to 'help manage' your child's tresses, kindly refuse and turn on your heels towards the nearest exit!

As read above the cons outweigh the Pro's with this treatment. In addition your child needs to learn about their natural beauty, trails and all. Your child will enjoy learning about how to care for their hair with you without the help of a relaxer. Enjoy those curls, kinks and coils and your child will love to also.

CONDITIONERS

Why condition the hair?

Conditioning afro/curly hair is one of the *single most important steps* in your child's whole hair care routine. Afro/curly hair is very fragile and almost always *naturally dry*. By adding conditioner to the hair, it is given a much-needed moisture-boost- that will help to keep it supple, healthy, shiny, soft and less prone to breakage. Unlike shampoo a good natural conditioner like our Cooler2cowash , will leave a barrier of much needed moisture and a detangling effect once rinsed off the hair. The hair cannot be conditioned enough!

Conditioner washing (Co-washing)

Afro hair and shampoos do not generally mix, this is why in the Shampoo tips it states- 'when shampooing your child's hair, ensure the shampoo stays on the scalp only, do not apply to the length of the hair, better still adopt the co-washing technique.

So what is *Co-washing*?

Co-washing is when a mild (daily use) moisturising conditioner like our 'Cooler2cowash is used to wash both the hair and scalp. You simply apply the conditioner in the same way you would a shampoo. Take a small amount in the palm of your hands and apply to the scalp, ensuring to massage well to dislodge dirt and grease. The great thing is, since your using conditioner you do not have to worry about the hair being stripped of its natural oils as the conditioner is good for the hair also so slather it on all over the hair too from root to tip. Simply rinse when completed. (remember to keep the hair sectioned and deal with one section at a time as described earlier to avoid tangles and knots!)

Deep Conditioning = Dreamy *Soft* Hair

It is super important to maintain a consistent routine of deep conditioning for your child's hair- whether Afro or Curly textured. Deep conditioning unlike a regular conditioner will strengthen the hair over time as most deep conditioning hair masks/conditioners contain a protein (hair strengthener) of some sort within their formulation. Popular proteins found in Deep conditioners include: *wheat protein, *oat protein, and *silk amino proteins. (Our Cooler2cowash can be used as a DEEP conditioner too as it contains *Silk protein)

How to Deep Condition Effectively:

1. After washing your child's hair in sections as described earlier- un-loose each section and apply a generous amount of your Deep conditioner.

2. Once applied to the section lightly re-plait it especially (if the hair is long enough/if not use banding bands) to eliminate tangles

3. Continue to do this until the whole head is covered

4. Next apply a plastic cap to the child's head and leave them to play or watch a DVD for at least 45 minutes,

5. Once the time is up- rinse the conditioner from the child's head- (use luke-warm to cool water for the final rinse) to reveal soft, silky deep conditioned hair- ready to be moisturised.

Hairducation Tip: Explain to your child- the conditioner is a curls best friend and to keep the hair healthy and strong we need to Deep condition and co-wash weekly)

SIMPLE, SAFE, EASY
'Soft Scalp Styles' for kids with Curls/Kinks:

OK, so we have covered the basics of Hairducation the ABC of it as I call it, including Hair Washing, Dealing with knots and How-to moisturise the hair and moisturising, but what about styling?

This chapter will focus on safe styling methods for your child's hair. I emphasise this phrase 'Soft Scalp Styling' or triple S. My role as a Hairducation expert has taken me around Europe delivering Hairducation workshops to parents in Milan, Paris, Brussels and London. What never surprises me is the fact that I have witnessed children with hair damage caused by bad styling choices all over Europe...this is very preventable with Hairducation!

What is a bad styling choice?
A bad styling choice is one that causes hair damage- most of the times actual hair loss! They include:

Tight thin cornrows
Bunches with elastics that are very tight ponytails (giving the appearance of a facelift)
Heavy or tight braid extensions
Hair weaves

How do we avoid such hair damage?
If you appreciate that your child's hair is attached to the scalp which when pulled too tightly over a period of time literally weeds the strand of hair out of its home- you will absorb the notion of 'Soft Scalp Styling'.

SAFE hair-styling Tools:
The following hair tools should be purchased to manage your child's hair:
The first thing you will need before you start styling is the correct tools! If you have straight hair or relaxed hair, the combs and brushes you use on your own hair- can cause damage to your child's curls or Afro hair!

I have always cornrowed my child's hair should I continue?
I would avoid the over-use of cornrows. They are not a '*Soft Scalp Style*'. More often than not they are done too tightly, leading to traction alopecia (hair loss) in children as young as 2! I have seen this. They can also thin-out the natural thickness of the child's hair when worn continuously.

Instead try single twists or braids. I love twists as they can be co-washed (**See conditioner tips**), and moisturised easily every day. Twists are soft on the scalp and allow the hair to grow freely.

No matter your styling choice- if the scalp is soft and not pulled on tightly to stress it the hair will remain healthy and grow well!

*Remember the hair is really delicate although it may appear to be very strong!

So what should I use?

- A seamless wide/tooth bone comb
- A quality plastic afro comb
- Soft boar brush- for smoothing the hair
- Soft metal free hair bands

Avoid at all costs:

Fine teeth combs
They tear and rip Afro hair out!

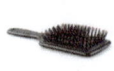
Brushes with hard plastic teeth
Are designed for straight hair!

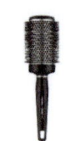
Round brushes with sharp spiked bristles
Are weapons of mass destruction!

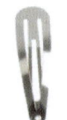
Hair clips with metal clasps
Pull and snag the hair causing breakage.

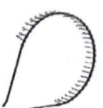
Hair/Alice bands with grips
Use the smooth based ones instead especially on Afro hair

Hairducation Tip:
'Only allow trusted hands in your child's hair'

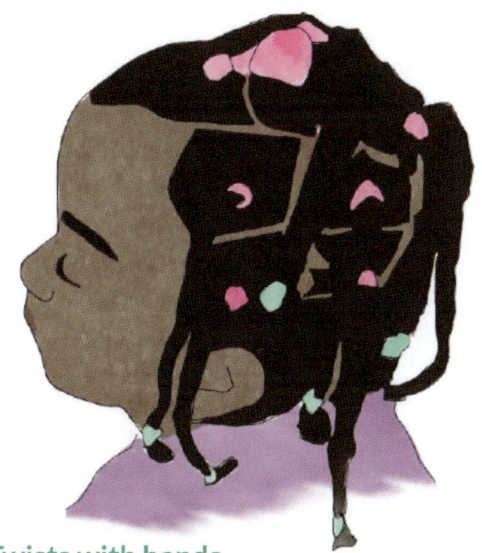

Twists with bands

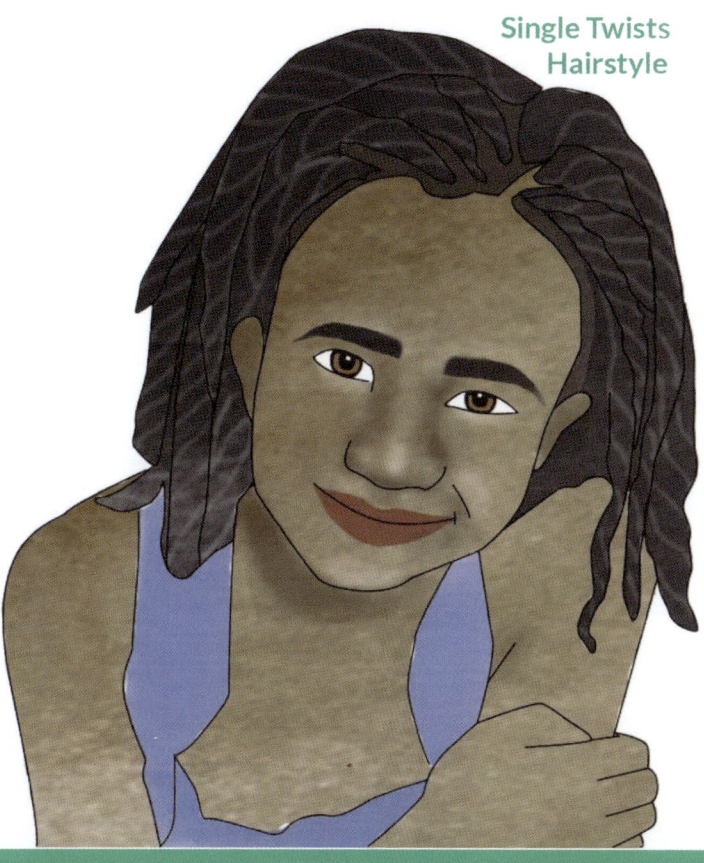

Single Twists Hairstyle

1. Start with freshly washed and conditioned and detangled hair- as described in the tips earlier,

2. Apply our Honey rain juice to the damp hair and part the hair into two sections by making a part with your comb from ear to ear horizontally, halfway down the head.

3. Put one half of the head- the front half in a hair band out of the way, as you will start from the back.

4. Starting at the back of the head near the left ear make another part from ear to ear horizontally about 2 inches up from the base of the head.

5. Apply a hair band to the hair not being used so it is out of your way.

6. Using your comb make a vertical part 2 inches from the left of the head all the way down so you have a square section of hair,

7. Again use a free hair band to move the remainding hair out of your way.

8 Using your fingers ensure the hair is detangled and before you will twist each section apply some of your twurly butter , sunlight curl crème or moisturiser of choice to the section of hair.

9. Using your boar bristle brush gently smooth the hair down, brushing right from the root to the tips of the hair.

10. Section that hair into two pieces and proceed to twist the half in your left hand across the half in your right hand.

11. Dependant on the hair texture you are working with you may need to use Twurly butter or Sunlight curl crème to smooth the twist and give it hold.

12. If the hair texture is very light the twist may not hold. In this case you
could place a metal/snag-free hair band at the base of the hair sectioned off and then maybe plait the hair instead and then place a hair-band at the end of the hair to prevent it unravelling.

13. Continue to do your box section 2-3 inch sized partings until the whole head is twisted.
Once the hair is covered at night with a satin scarf or bonnet, the hair will not get overly dry, and the style will last longer.

14. Spritz the twists/plaits every day or other day with your Honey rain juice, to prevent dryness.

15. Continue to do this to each row of hair until completed. You may then style the twists or leave them loose.

PRODUCT GUIDE

If you do not share the same hair type as your child for example you are a white mum and you have **mixed children or you are a black mum with mixed children or black children who have a different hair type to your own, Fear not!** This mini guide to the right products will help! Natural Hair Products are always far better for Mixed, Curly and afro hair, in fact this is true for any hair type.

Natural products have a natural affinity to the hair and just make the hair feel and look healthier. Kinki Coili Kurli products are natural and organic and were created by me in my kitchen as I could find no natural products in my local beauty supply shop to suit my daughter's frizzy curly hair. In addition as she was born with 6 food allergies and suffered with eczema so I wanted products I used to be natural and not full of chemical as they were going onto her hair and scalp.

After much trial and error and many nights alone in my kitchen I have managed to create a range of products for children that give the amazing results! Check out the products below, they suit all Curly, Wavy, Coily and Kinky hair textures- they nourish without being greasy!

Kinki Coili Curli
Natural haircare for kids with curls

Hairducation Tip: Avoid hair grease and hair products with chemicals, like mineral oil, petroleum and lanolin! keep it natural

The Honey Rain Juice
Use this to detangle knots/Spritz hair daily/sandwich moisture

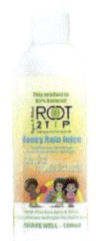

Cool Mint Curls Cleanser (SLS free)
Use to shampoo the hair and scalp

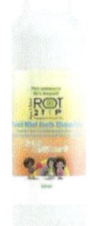

Heaven's Hair Milk
Use on baby Hair, or step 2 in the Sandwich moisture method, also for light daily moisture on fine hair

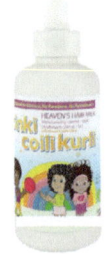

Cooler2Cowash Conditioner
Use to Deep condition, and Co-wash the hair

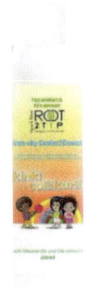

Sunlight Curl creme
Apply on damp hair to define curls and moisturise hair

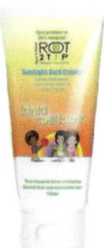

Star-Shine Hair & Scalp Oil
Use to oil and massage the scalp /use on hair if needed

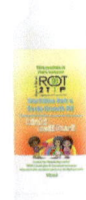

INVEST

'In these essential hair care items for your child's hair!'

Wide Tooth Comb

Use to detangle after using hands!

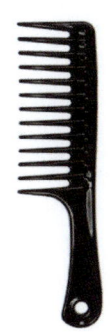

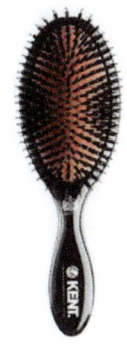

Soft Boar Brush

Use this for smoothing the hair into place when styling.

KCK Co-wash Conditioner

Use this to cleanse curls and **deep condition strands**

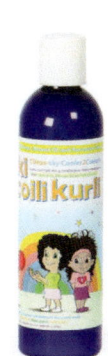

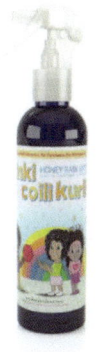

Honey Rain Juice

This daily leave-in conditioner/ detangler is great for Afro/ Curly hair! and 98 its 98.5% natural too.

Hair Bands

Use these to style hair **safely- not tightly** remember the triple S rule, **(Soft Scalp Styling)**

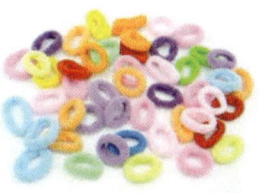

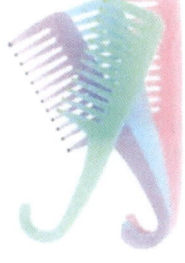

Shower Comb

Grab yourself a great shower comb, it is soft on the hair and great for wet combing.

Satin Bonnet

This is for older children to protect their hair whilst sleeping.

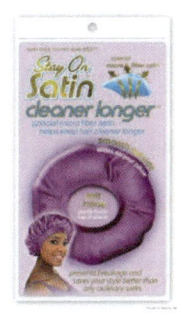

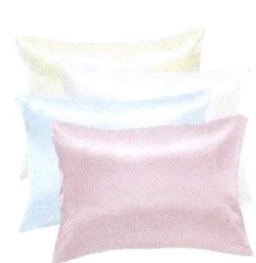

Satin Pillow Case

Use this to protect curls/ kinks from drying out and breakage

FAQ's on everything Kiddy Hair!

MY CHILD HAS JUST STARTED SWIMMING- PLEASE HELP:

Chlorine is bad for Afro and Mixed race hair- it makes the hair very dry and that will lead to breakage.

1 Apply Extra Virgin Olive oil or our Cooler2cowash conditioner to the child's hair, this will act as a barrier to the chlorine water. Do this the NIGHT BEFORE SWIMMING

2 If your child has very thick hair, style the hair in a banding style, twists, or loose plaits. Make it easy for them to apply the swimming cap if swimming at school.

3 Always wear a swim cap- Invest in a large swimming cap for long hair, if your child has lots of hair! Ensure they wear it!

4 After swimming -rinse your child's hair then wash with a mild shampoo then follow up with a 5 minute conditioner treatment. (IF the hair is in twists do not loose them out do it whilst hair is braided/twisted it works!)

HOW OFTEN DO I MOISTURISE MY CHILDS HAIR?

Moisturise the child's hair every day, it is as essential as brushing your teeth and teach your child this too. Mixed and afro hair is always dry! Use something like our Honey-rain juice, Heaven's hair milk or Sunlight Curl crème to give the hair a boost of hydration. Let them do it themselves- Hairducation is power!

SHOULD I BLOW-DRY MY CHILDS HAIR?

Try to limit blow dry usage on kids hair- instead use a t-shirt to dry the hair with, gently squeeze the water out of the hair, apply your moisturiser then style and let it air-dry. (Your child will not catch a cold!

MY CHILD SCREAMS WHEN SHE HAS HER HAIR DONE AT THE SALON: WHY?

If you take a child to a salon to have the hair braided or cornrowed and they scream in pain- its because IT HURTS!! please listen and do not take them there again! Many salons braid hair too tightly, brush/comb hair roughly all of which will cause damage to the hairline and your child's hair overall.

HOW OFTEN SHOULD I COMB/BRUSH THROUGH MY CHILDS HAIR?

My rule is generally- No Combs Allowed!

As Afro and Mixed race hair is very fragile, sadly, children often lose handfuls of 'good hair' through the act of 'daily brushing' (fine for straight hair not for curls/kinks!). Keep brushing to 'hair wash days', or when the hair is drenched in our Cooler2Co-wash conditioner or sprayed with Honey rain Juice.

> **Sal say's:**
> Stick to the rules - if you take your child to family/friends ensure they respect the hair rules you follow for your child!- remember one bad blow-dry or comb-out can ruin years of tender hair care!

HELP: MY CHILDS HAIR IS NOT GROWING!

I hear this comment all the time- truthfully everyone alive is growing hair continually- however it may be your hair routine that is preventing you seeing the growth I grew my daughters Afro hair to waist-length by age 4 by doing the following:

- Only doing Low manipulation styles- twists, single braids, banding, loose hair-

- Let the hair be messy! Again styling the hair daily –leads to breakage on afro and mixed hair leave styles in for a week 2 weeks at a time!

- Eliminating a dry scalp- plants do not grow in dry soil! Oil and massage the scalp weekly with our StarShine Hair& Scalp Growth oil- 100% Natural! (use a natural oil on the scalp always!) massage feeds the roots under the scalp that produce hair!

- No Blow-drying air-dry the hair instead, excess wet without a heat protectant) grease will not protect!) Leads to damaged hair that breaks like straw!

- Dry hair- Daily Moisturising and regular co-washing and deep conditioning will lead to longer hair

- BE PATIENT and give TLC- the best way to see your child's hair grow well is to give it time and stick to a simple regime.

This essential guide is the first published book from the ROOT2TiP Hairducation Academy. It has been written with love especially for parents/carers who have children with Mixed race and Afro hair textures, however the rules will also apply to those with just frizzy curls too! For many years parents have struggled not knowing what to do to their children's hair. We want to turn hair day tears into cheers!

We have broken down haircare into easy to learn sections that will soon turn you into a hair care expert with practice and patience.

The Hairducation in this great guide will break down the simple steps needed to correctly care for your child's hair, whilst at the same time teach them good hair rules also.

It's time to create Happy Hair days at home!!

Hairducation is Power!

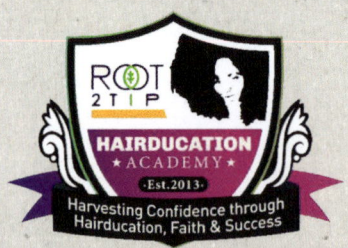

Stay in touch with the Hairducation Academy

The Hairducation Academy is the UK's best resource for hair that is not straight. Visit our website and check out the new additions to our book shop, other great tips, our blog, style gallery, Hairducation event/Workshop dates, Cool kid's photo shoots, and much much more.

Visit our website :

www.hairducation-academy.org.uk

Check out and purchase Kinki Coili Kurli natural hair products here :

www.root2tip.com

Stay in touch with us on social media :

@ root2tip

Check out and subscribe to the :
Heavenberry Hairshow 4 kids

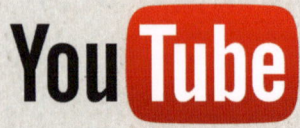

Printed in Great Britain
by Amazon